ILEOSTOMY DIET COOKBOOK FOR BEGINNERS

An Ultimate Guide to manage ileostomy with easy-to-prepare recipes, right diet modification and activity

MELINDA JAYDEN

Copyright © 2024 by Melinda Jayden

All rights reserved. No part of this publication may be reproduced, distributed, or transmitted in any form or by any means, including photocopying, recording, or other electronic or mechanical methods, without the prior written permission of the publisher, except in the case of brief quotations embodied in critical reviews and certain other noncommercial uses permitted by copyright law.

TABLE OF CONTENT

INTRODUCTION..5
CHAPTER 1: UNDERSTANDING ILEOSTOMY..6
   1.1 What it is and how it affects Digestion...6
   1.2 Importance of Diet in Managing Ileostomy..7
   1.3 Tips for Successful Diet Management with an Ileostomy............................8

CHAPTER 2: FOUNDATIONS OF AN ILEOSTOMY-FRIENDLY DIET............9
   2.1 Restricted Foods..9
   2.2 Importance of Fiber and Ways to Incorporate It..12

CHAPTER 3: UNDERSTANDING LOW-FIBER AND LOW-RESIDUE DIET..13
   3.1 Reasons for Following a Low-Fiber Diet..13
   3.2 Important Components of a Low-Fiber Diet...14
   3.3 Practical Tips for Low-Fiber and Low-Residue Eating with an Ileostomy...........16

CHAPTER 4: MEAL PLANNING FOR ILEOSTOMY PATIENTS...................18
   4.1 Creating Balanced Meals..18
   4.2 Portion Control and Timing of Meals...19
   4.3 Strategies for Meal Prep and Quick Snacks on the Go..............................20

CHAPTER 5: WHAT TO CONSIDER IN AN ILEOSTOMY DIET...................21
   5.1 Managing Dehydration...21
   5.2 Handling Gas and Odor: Foods to Minimize Odor and Bloating.............23
   5.3 Addressing Nutrient Absorption Issues and Vitamin Deficiencies...........24

CHAPTER 6: ILEOSTOMY-FRIENDLY DIET..25
BREAKFAST RECIPES...25
   Low-Fiber Pancakes..25
   Banana Oat Pancakes...26
   Egg and Spinach Muffins...27
   Greek Yogurt Parfait..27
   Smoothie Bowl..28
   Scrambled Eggs with Avocado..28
   Quinoa Breakfast Bowl..29

Cottage Cheese with Peach Slices..29
Turkey and Cheese Roll-Ups...30
Almond Butter and Banana Toast..30
Yogurt and Berry Smoothie..31
Egg White Omelett..31
Cinnamon Apple Porridge..32
Smoked Salmon and Cream Cheese Bagel...32
Rice Cake with Peanut Butter and Sliced Banana.....................................33
Mango Coconut Yogurt Bowl...33
Egg and Cheese Breakfast Quesadilla...34
Vanilla Protein Shake..34
Cheddar Cheese and Tomato Toast...35
Blueberry Almond Smoothie...35

LUNCH RECIPES..**36**
Quinoa Salad with Grilled Chicken...36
Turkey and Avocado Wrap...36
Salmon and Quinoa Bowl...37
Egg Salad Lettuce Wraps..38
Tuna and White Bean Salad..39
Chicken and Vegetable Stir-Fry..39
Mashed Sweet Potatoes with Grilled Shrimp...40
Spinach and Feta Omelette...40
Baked Cod with Steamed Vegetables..41
Turkey and Vegetable Soup...41
Shredded Chicken and Brown Rice Bowl..42
Tofu and Vegetable Stir-Fry...42
Lentil Soup with Spinach..43
Grilled Vegetable Salad...43
Miso Soup with Tofu and Seaweed..44

ASIAN RECIPES..**45**
Steamed Fish with Ginger and Scallions...45
Vegetable Stir-Fry..45
Ginger Chicken Congee..46
Japanese Omelette (Tamagoyaki)..46
Rice Noodle Soup..47

PORTUGUESE RECIPES... 48
Bacalhau à Brás (Portuguese Salt Cod Hash)................................48
Caldo Verde (Portuguese Green Soup)...48
Grilled Sardines...49
Portuguese Chicken and Rice..49
Portuguese Custard Tarts (Pastéis de Nata)..................................50

SPANISH RECIPES... 51
Spanish Tortilla (Tortilla Española)..51
Gazpacho..51
Spanish Rice with Shrimp..52
Patatas Bravas..52
Spanish Chicken Paella..53

ITALIAN RECIPES.. 54
Caprese Salad...54
Pasta Primavera...54
Chicken Piccata..55
Minestrone Soup..55
Tiramisu...56

BONUS.. 57
28 days MEAL PLAN..57

CONCLUSION.. 60

INTRODUCTION

Living with an ileostomy presents its fair share of challenges, both physical and emotional. From managing output consistency and preventing skin irritation to getting through social situations and maintaining a positive body image, there's no shortage of obstacles to overcome. However, with the right knowledge, support, and mindset, individuals with an ileostomy can lead full, active lives and thrive in spite of any challenges they may face.

An ileostomy is a surgical procedure in which a portion of the small intestine, known as the ileum, is brought to the surface of the abdomen to form a stoma. This stoma serves as an alternative route for waste to leave the body when the natural digestive process is interrupted or compromised. Ileostomies are commonly performed to treat conditions such as inflammatory bowel disease (IBD), colorectal cancer, diverticulitis, or trauma to the digestive tract.

One of the most common concerns for people with an ileostomy is managing output consistency and preventing leakage. Because waste passes through the small intestine more quickly than usual, output from an ileostomy tends to be more liquid and frequent. To manage this, individuals must wear an ostomy pouching system—a specialized bag that collects waste and adheres to the skin around the stoma. Proper fitting and care of the pouching system are essential for preventing leaks, skin irritation, and other complications.

This brings us to the primary purpose of this book: **ILEOSTOMY DIET COOKBOOK FOR BEGINNERS**. In the following sections, we will explore the complexities of dietary management for individuals with an ileostomy, analyzing the foods to enjoy, foods to limit or avoid, and successful strategies for improving nutrition and hydration. From understanding the basics of digestion to mastering the art of meal planning and recipe modification, we will provide you with the knowledge, tools, and resources needed to navigate the world of nutrition and diet with ease and confidence.

Incorporating adequate protein into your diet is essential for supporting healing, maintaining muscle mass, and promoting overall health and vitality. Good sources of protein for ileostomy patients include lean meats, poultry, fish, eggs, dairy products, tofu, legumes, and nuts and seeds. Aim to include protein with each meal and snack to help keep you feeling satisfied and energized throughout the day.

CHAPTER 1: UNDERSTANDING ILEOSTOMY

1.1 What it is and how it affects Digestion

An ileostomy is a surgical procedure that involves the creation of an opening, called a stoma, in the abdomen through which a portion of the small intestine, known as the ileum, is then brought to the surface of the skin. This surgical intervention is typically performed as a treatment for various medical conditions, such as inflammatory bowel disease (IBD), colorectal cancer, familial adenomatous polyposis (FAP), or trauma to the digestive system.

The creation of an ileostomy fundamentally alters the normal digestive process. In a healthy individual, the small intestine absorbs water and nutrients from the food as it passes through, while waste products continue their journey through the large intestine, where water is further absorbed, and stool is formed. However, with an ileostomy, the usual route for waste elimination is bypassed, leading to changes in bowel function and digestion.

Because the contents of the small intestine, including digestive enzymes and bile salts, are now discharged directly through the stoma, there are implications for digestion and nutrient absorption. Without the large intestine's role in absorbing excess water and electrolytes, stool output tends to be more liquid and frequent. Additionally, certain nutrients, such as water-soluble vitamins and electrolytes, may be excreted in higher amounts, potentially leading to deficiencies if not managed appropriately.

There are various reasons why an ileostomy might be recommended. Some of the most common conditions prompting surgery include:

Ulcerative colitis: This chronic inflammatory bowel disease (IBD) causes inflammation and ulcers in the colon lining. In severe cases, the colon may need to be removed.
Crohn's disease: Another IBD, Crohn's disease can affect any part of the digestive tract, including the colon. Surgery might be necessary if medication fails to control the inflammation or complications arise.
Colon cancer: When cancerous cells are found in the colon, surgical removal of the affected portion – sometimes the entire colon – is necessary.
Diverticulitis: This condition involves inflammation and infection in pouches that form in the colon wall. If severe or recurring, surgery to remove the diseased section might be needed.

1.2 Importance of Diet in Managing Ileostomy

Diet plays an important role in managing an ileostomy effectively. Since the digestive process is altered following surgery, it is essential to make dietary adjustments to minimize complications and optimize health outcomes. Proper nutrition can help individuals with an ileostomy maintain their energy levels, prevent dehydration, and mitigate the risk of nutrient deficiencies.

One of the primary concerns for individuals with an ileostomy is maintaining adequate hydration. With increased fluid loss through the stoma, there is a higher risk of dehydration, which can lead to symptoms such as fatigue, dizziness, and electrolyte imbalances. Therefore, consuming sufficient fluids, such as water, herbal teas, and electrolyte-replenishing drinks, is essential for preventing dehydration and maintaining hydration levels.

Furthermore, dietary modifications may be necessary to manage the consistency and frequency of stool output. Certain foods, such as high-fiber fruits and vegetables, whole grains, and seeds, can contribute to bulkier stools and increased transit time, which may exacerbate symptoms such as diarrhea and gas production. Conversely, a low-fiber diet consisting of easily digestible foods, such as white rice, bananas, cooked vegetables, and lean proteins, may help alleviate these symptoms and promote greater stool control.

In addition to managing hydration and stool consistency, diet plays a crucial role in preventing nutrient deficiencies commonly associated with ileostomy surgery. Since the absorption of certain nutrients, such as vitamin B12, iron, and calcium, may be impaired following surgery, it is essential to focus on nutrient-dense foods and, in some cases, consider supplementation to meet nutritional needs adequately.

1.3 Tips for Successful Diet Management with an Ileostomy

Stay Hydrated: Drink plenty of fluids throughout the day to prevent dehydration. Aim for at least eight glasses of water daily, and consider consuming electrolyte-replenishing drinks to maintain electrolyte balance.

Monitor Stool Output: Pay attention to the consistency and frequency of stool output, as this can indicate whether dietary modifications are necessary. Keep track of food intake and bowel movements to identify any patterns or triggers.

Follow a Low-Fiber Diet: Initially, focus on consuming foods that are low in fiber to minimize digestive discomfort and promote better stool control. Opt for cooked vegetables, white bread, pasta, and peeled fruits to reduce fiber intake.

Chew Food Thoroughly: Take your time to chew food thoroughly before swallowing, as this can aid digestion and minimize the risk of blockages or obstructions in the digestive tract.

Limit Gas-Producing Foods: Avoid foods that are known to cause gas and bloating, such as beans, cabbage, onions, and carbonated beverages. Opt for smaller, more frequent meals to reduce the likelihood of excessive gas production.

Incorporate Nutrient-Dense Foods: Focus on consuming nutrient-dense foods to meet your body's nutritional needs. Include sources of lean protein, such as poultry, fish, and tofu, as well as fruits, vegetables, and dairy products fortified with calcium and vitamin D.

Consider Supplementation: Consult with a healthcare professional or registered dietitian to determine whether supplementation is necessary to address any potential nutrient deficiencies. Vitamin and mineral supplements may be recommended to ensure adequate nutrient intake.

Seek Support: Joining a support group or seeking guidance from a healthcare provider specializing in ostomy care can provide valuable information and support for managing diet and lifestyle adjustments following ileostomy surgery.

CHAPTER 2: FOUNDATIONS OF AN ILEOSTOMY-FRIENDLY DIET

2.1 Restricted Foods

Living with an ileostomy can bring about significant changes in one's dietary habits and lifestyle. Whether you've recently undergone ileostomy surgery or you're exploring options to support someone who has, understanding the foundations of an ileostomy-friendly diet is crucial for maintaining health, managing symptoms, and ensuring overall well-being. When adapting to life with an ileostomy, it's essential to be mindful of the foods you consume. Certain foods can help prevent complications and promote better digestion, while others may exacerbate symptoms or lead to discomfort.

Here's a breakdown of foods to include and avoid:

Foods to Include:
Low-fiber fruits and vegetables: Opt for fruits and vegetables that are easy to digest, such as bananas, peeled apples, cooked carrots, and squash. These choices provide essential vitamins and minerals without overwhelming the digestive system.

Lean proteins: Incorporate lean sources of protein like chicken, fish, eggs, and tofu into your meals. Protein is essential for tissue repair and overall health.

Refined grains: Choose refined grains like white rice, white bread, and pasta over their whole grain counterparts. These options are gentler on the digestive system and less likely to cause blockages.

Dairy alternatives: If lactose intolerance is an issue, consider dairy alternatives like almond milk, soy milk, or lactose-free dairy products to meet calcium needs.

Nutrient-dense foods: Focus on nutrient-dense foods such as nuts, seeds, nut butter, and avocados to ensure you're getting essential vitamins and minerals.

Foods to Avoid:

High-fiber foods: Steer clear of high-fiber foods like raw vegetables, fruits with skins or seeds, whole grains, and legumes. These can be difficult to digest and may increase the risk of blockages.

Gas-producing foods: Minimize consumption of gas-producing foods such as beans, cabbage, broccoli, and carbonated beverages, as they can cause discomfort and bloating. Tough or stringy meats: Avoid tough cuts of meat and opt for tender cuts instead to prevent digestive issues.

Spicy and acidic foods: Limit intake of spicy foods, citrus fruits, tomatoes, and vinegar, as they may irritate the digestive tract and cause discomfort.

High-fat foods: Reduce consumption of high-fat foods like fried foods, creamy sauces, and fatty cuts of meat, as they can contribute to diarrhea and malabsorption.

Balancing Nutrition: Vitamins, Minerals, and Fluid Intake
Maintaining proper nutrition is essential for individuals with an ileostomy to support healing, prevent deficiencies, and promote overall health.

Here are some strategies for balancing nutrition:

Multivitamin supplementation: Consider taking a daily multivitamin to ensure you're meeting your nutritional needs, especially if your diet is limited.

Focus on hydration: Stay hydrated by drinking plenty of fluids throughout the day. Aim for at least eight glasses of water daily, and avoid excessive consumption of caffeinated or alcoholic beverages, as they can contribute to dehydration.

Monitor electrolytes: Keep an eye on your electrolyte levels, particularly sodium, potassium, and magnesium. Electrolyte imbalances can occur more easily with an ileostomy due to increased fluid loss, so incorporating electrolyte-rich foods like bananas, potatoes, and sports drinks can be beneficial.

Incorporate vitamin-rich foods: Include foods rich in vitamins A, C, D, E, and K in your diet to support immune function, wound healing, and overall health. Citrus fruits, leafy greens, dairy products, eggs, and fortified cereals are excellent sources of essential vitamins.

Consider calcium supplementation: Since calcium absorption may be compromised with an ileostomy, talk to your healthcare provider about whether calcium supplementation is necessary to maintain bone health.

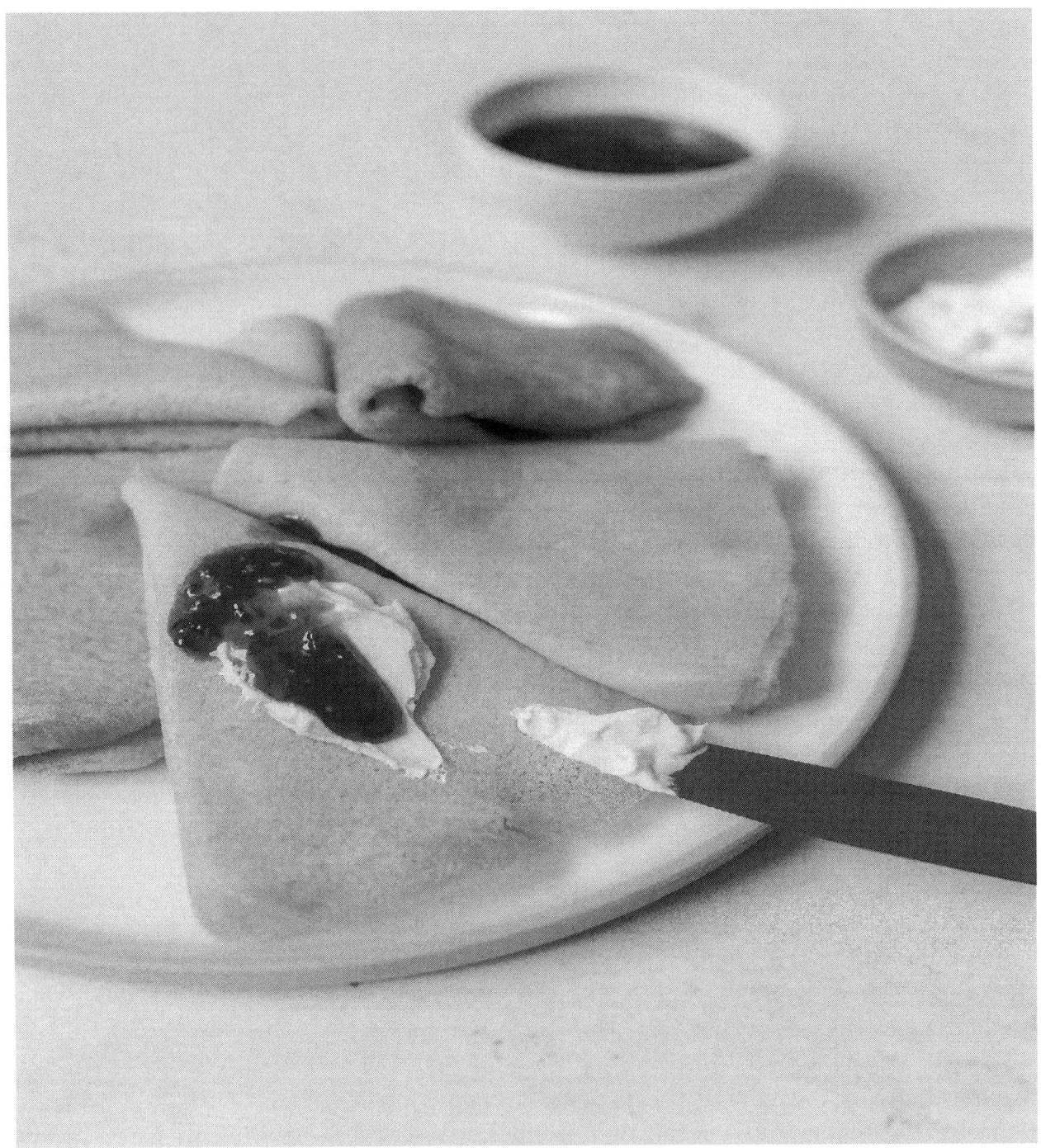

2.2 Importance of Fiber and Ways to Incorporate It

While a high-fiber diet is typically recommended for digestive health, individuals with an ileostomy may need to approach fiber intake differently. Fiber can be beneficial in regulating bowel movements, preventing constipation, and promoting overall digestive health. However, too much fiber can lead to blockages and discomfort for those with an ileostomy.

Here are some ways to incorporate fiber into an ileostomy-friendly diet:

Start slow: Gradually introduce fiber-rich foods into your diet and monitor how your body responds. Begin with small portions and increase gradually to assess tolerance.

Choose soluble fiber: Focus on incorporating soluble fiber sources such as oatmeal, barley, psyllium husk, and flaxseeds into your meals. Soluble fiber dissolves in water and forms a gel-like substance, which can help regulate bowel movements without causing blockages.

Cook vegetables: Cooked vegetables are generally easier to digest than raw ones. Steam, boil, or roast vegetables to make them more tender and digestible.

Puree or blend fruits and vegetables: If you have difficulty digesting whole fruits and vegetables, try pureeing or blending them into smoothies or soups for easier consumption.

Consider fiber supplements: Talk to your healthcare provider about whether fiber supplements such as methylcellulose or psyllium husk are appropriate for you. These supplements can help increase fiber intake without causing digestive issues.

Incorporating these strategies into your daily routine can help you maintain a balanced and nourishing diet while living with an ileostomy. Remember to listen to your body, work closely with your healthcare team, and make adjustments as needed to support your unique dietary needs and preferences. With time and experimentation, you can find a diet that promotes optimal health and well-being while managing the challenges of life with an ileostomy.

CHAPTER 3: UNDERSTANDING LOW-FIBER AND LOW-RESIDUE DIET

3.1 Reasons for Following a Low-Fiber Diet

A low-fiber diet, also known as a low-residue diet, involves reducing the intake of foods high in dietary fiber. Fiber is the indigestible part of plant foods that adds bulk to the stool and aids in bowel movements. While fiber is generally beneficial for digestive health, there are certain medical conditions and situations where a low-fiber diet may be necessary or recommended.

Gastrointestinal Disorders: Individuals with certain gastrointestinal disorders such as Crohn's disease, ulcerative colitis, diverticulitis, or irritable bowel syndrome (IBS) may benefit from a low-fiber diet. High-fiber foods can exacerbate symptoms such as abdominal pain, bloating, and diarrhea in these conditions.

Pre- and Post-Surgical Needs: Before certain medical procedures or surgeries involving the gastrointestinal tract, healthcare providers may recommend a low-fiber diet to reduce the volume and bulk of stool, making it easier to manage and reducing the risk of complications during and after the procedure.

Symptom Management: Some people experience gastrointestinal symptoms such as gas, cramping, or diarrhea when consuming high-fiber foods. A low-fiber diet can help alleviate these symptoms and improve overall comfort.

Dental or Swallowing Issues: Individuals with dental problems or difficulty swallowing may find it challenging to consume high-fiber foods. In such cases, a low-fiber diet can provide relief and ensure adequate nutrition without causing discomfort.

3.2 Important Components of a Low-Fiber Diet

Limiting High-Fiber Foods: The primary focus of a low-fiber diet is to reduce or eliminate foods that are high in fiber. This includes whole grains, legumes, nuts, seeds, fruits with skins and seeds, and vegetables with tough skins or seeds.

Choosing Refined and Processed Foods: Refined grains and processed foods are typically lower in fiber compared to their whole counterparts. Opt for white bread, white rice, refined pasta, and processed cereals instead of whole grain options.

Cooking Methods: Certain cooking methods can help make high-fiber foods more digestible. For example, peeling fruits and vegetables, removing seeds from fruits, and cooking vegetables until they are soft can reduce their fiber content.

Focusing on Low-Fiber Alternatives: While following a low-fiber diet, it's important to include nutrient-rich foods that are gentle on the digestive system. This includes lean proteins, dairy products, eggs, tender cooked vegetables, and well-cooked grains such as white rice.

Essential Considerations for an Ileostomy Diet

Reducing Fiber Intake: Unlike individuals with a fully intact digestive tract, those with an ileostomy must be cautious about consuming high-fiber foods. Fiber, particularly insoluble fiber found in fruits, vegetables, whole grains, and nuts, can be difficult to digest and may lead to blockages or irritation around the stoma. Therefore, a low-fiber diet is often recommended to minimize the risk of complications.

Managing Residue: Residue refers to undigested food particles that pass through the digestive system and can contribute to stool bulk. Since individuals with an ileostomy have a shorter transit time for waste elimination, minimizing residue is essential to prevent ostomy bag leakage, irritation, or discomfort. This involves choosing foods that are easily digestible and produce minimal waste.

Balancing Fluid and Electrolytes: With the colon bypassed, the body may experience increased fluid and electrolyte losses through the ileostomy output. Dehydration and electrolyte imbalances are common concerns, especially during periods of high output or in hot weather. Therefore, staying adequately hydrated and replenishing electrolytes through dietary sources or supplements is crucial for maintaining optimal health.

Ensuring Nutritional Adequacy: Despite the need to limit certain foods, it's essential for individuals with an ileostomy to obtain sufficient nutrients to support healing, energy levels, and overall well-being. This requires careful planning and attention to nutrient-rich foods that are gentle on the digestive system and easily absorbed.

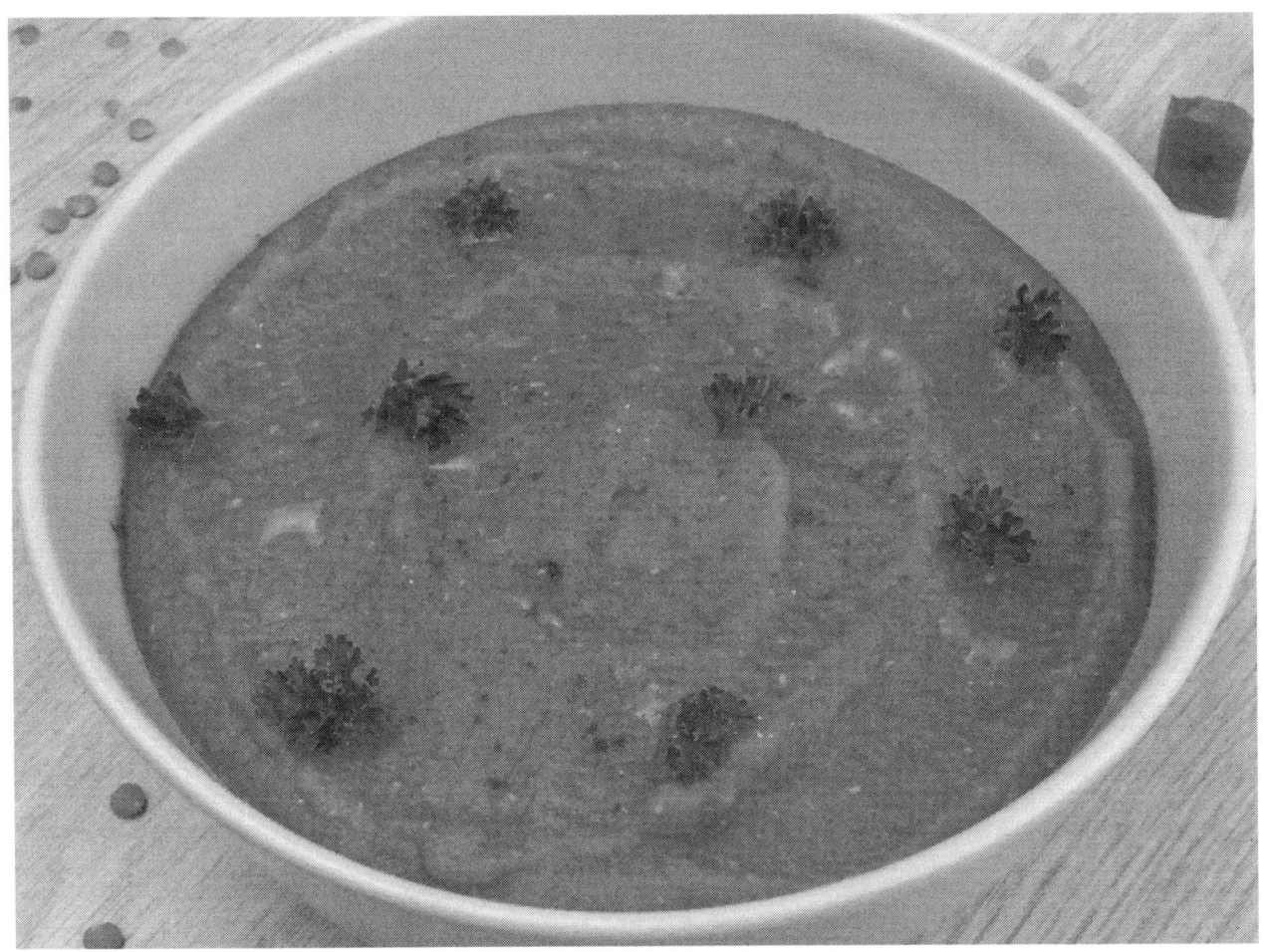

3.3 Practical Tips for Low-Fiber and Low-Residue Eating with an Ileostomy

Choose Refined Grains: Opt for refined grains such as white bread, white rice, and refined pasta instead of whole grain varieties, which contain higher amounts of fiber. These processed grains are easier to digest and less likely to contribute to ostomy output.

Cook Fruits and Vegetables: While raw fruits and vegetables are rich in nutrients, they can be challenging for individuals with an ileostomy to tolerate due to their high fiber content. Instead, cook or steam fruits and vegetables to soften them and make them more digestible. Removing seeds, skins, and fibrous parts can further reduce residue.

Include Lean Proteins: Focus on incorporating lean proteins such as poultry, fish, eggs, and tofu into your diet. These protein sources are low in fiber and residue, making them well-suited for individuals with an ileostomy.

Limit Gas-Producing Foods: Certain foods, such as beans, cabbage, onions, and carbonated beverages, can increase gas production and lead to bloating or discomfort. Minimize or avoid these gas-producing foods to reduce the risk of ostomy bag ballooning or leakage.

Stay Hydrated: Drink plenty of fluids throughout the day to prevent dehydration and maintain adequate hydration levels. Water, herbal teas, and electrolyte-rich beverages can help replace lost fluids and electrolytes due to ileostomy output.

Monitor Ostomy Output: Pay attention to the consistency, color, and frequency of your ileostomy output, as these can indicate your digestive health and hydration status. If you notice significant changes or abnormalities, consult with your healthcare provider for guidance.

Addressing Common Concerns and Challenges

Nutritional Deficiencies: One concern with a low-fiber and low-residue diet is the potential for nutrient deficiencies, particularly in vitamins, minerals, and fiber. To mitigate this risk, consider working with a registered dietitian who can help you plan balanced meals and recommend appropriate supplements if needed.

Impact on Bowel Function: Some individuals worry that following a low-fiber diet may lead to constipation or irregular bowel movements. However, with an ileostomy, the primary goal is to reduce the risk of blockages or complications, rather than promoting regularity through fiber intake. Adequate hydration, gentle physical activity, and monitoring of ileostomy output can help maintain bowel function.

Social and Emotional Impact: Adapting to dietary restrictions imposed by an ileostomy can have social and emotional implications, such as feeling limited in food choices or self-conscious about ostomy bag management in social settings. It's important to seek support from healthcare professionals, ostomy support groups, or mental health professionals to address these concerns and develop coping strategies.

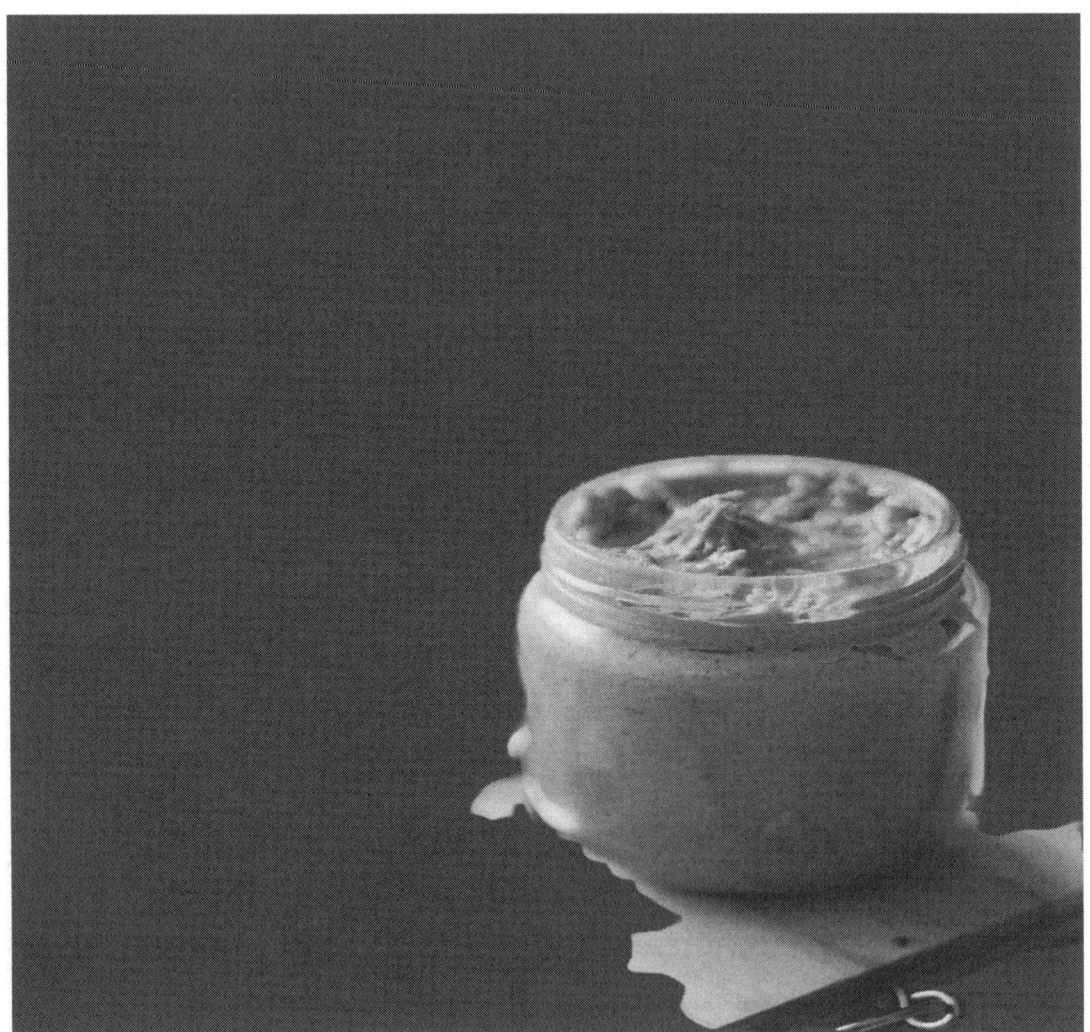

CHAPTER 4: MEAL PLANNING FOR ILEOSTOMY PATIENTS

4.1 Creating Balanced Meals

Living with an ileostomy can present unique challenges when it comes to meal planning. It's essential to maintain balanced nutrition while also considering factors such as portion control, timing of meals, and convenience. In this chapter, we'll explore strategies for creating balanced meals, managing portion sizes, and preparing quick snacks on the go for ileostomy patients.

Balanced nutrition is important for ileostomy patients to support overall health and well-being. When planning meals, it's essential to include a variety of nutrient-rich foods to ensure adequate intake of protein, carbohydrates, and fats.

Proteins: Protein is essential for tissue repair and maintaining muscle mass, especially important for individuals recovering from surgery. Good sources of protein for ileostomy patients include lean meats such as chicken, turkey, and fish. Plant-based options like beans, lentils, tofu, and quinoa are also excellent choices. It's essential to choose lean protein sources to minimize the risk of stoma-related complications.

Carbohydrates: Carbohydrates provide the body with energy and should be included in every meal. Opt for complex carbohydrates like whole grains, fruits, and vegetables, which provide fiber and essential nutrients. Avoid refined carbohydrates and sugary foods, as they can lead to digestive discomfort and may exacerbate ileostomy symptoms.

Fats: Healthy fats are essential for nutrient absorption and hormone production. Choose sources of unsaturated fats such as avocados, nuts, seeds, and olive oil. Limit saturated and trans fats found in fried foods, processed snacks, and fatty meats, as they can contribute to inflammation and digestive issues.

4.2 Portion Control and Timing of Meals

Portion control is crucial for ileostomy patients to prevent digestive discomfort and maintain optimal weight. Eating smaller, more frequent meals throughout the day can help prevent overloading the digestive system and minimize the risk of stoma-related complications.

Smaller Meals: Aim for 4-6 smaller meals per day rather than 3 large meals. This approach can help prevent bloating, gas, and diarrhea, common concerns for ileostomy patients.

Balanced Portions: When planning meals, aim to fill half of your plate with fruits and vegetables, one-quarter with lean protein, and one-quarter with whole grains or starchy vegetables. This balanced approach ensures you're getting a variety of nutrients without overloading your system.

Timing: Pay attention to the timing of your meals and snacks, especially in relation to physical activity and medication. Eating a small snack before exercise can provide energy without causing digestive discomfort, while waiting at least 2 hours after meals before engaging in strenuous activity can help prevent issues like dehydration and bowel obstruction.

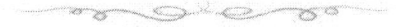

4.3 Strategies for Meal Prep and Quick Snacks on the Go

Meal prep and quick snacks are essential for ileostomy patients, especially when faced with busy schedules or traveling. Here are some strategies to make meal planning and snacking easier:

Pre-cut and Pre-packaged Foods: Wash, chop, and portion out fruits, vegetables, and other snacks in advance. Store them in convenient containers or resealable bags for easy access throughout the week.

Protein-Packed Snacks: Keep protein-rich snacks on hand, such as hard-boiled eggs, Greek yogurt, cheese sticks, or protein bars. These portable options provide energy and help maintain muscle mass.

Homemade Convenience Foods: Prepare homemade versions of convenience foods like granola bars, energy bites, or trail mix using nutritious ingredients like oats, nuts, seeds, and dried fruit. This allows you to control the ingredients and avoid additives or preservatives that may aggravate digestive symptoms.

Hydration: Stay hydrated by carrying a water bottle with you throughout the day. Sip fluids regularly to prevent dehydration, which can worsen ileostomy symptoms.

Emergency Snack Kit: Create an emergency snack kit containing non-perishable items like crackers, nut butter packets, rice cakes, and dried fruit. Keep it in your bag or car for quick access when hunger strikes.

Meal planning for ileostomy patients involves creating balanced meals, managing portion sizes, and preparing convenient snacks for on-the-go. By prioritizing nutrient-rich foods, practicing portion control, and implementing meal prep strategies, individuals with an ileostomy can enjoy a varied and satisfying diet while supporting their overall health and well-being.

CHAPTER 5: WHAT TO CONSIDER IN AN ILEOSTOMY DIET

Living with an ileostomy comes with its own set of challenges, particularly when it comes to managing diet and nutrition. In this chapter, we'll look into some special considerations for individuals with an ileostomy, including managing dehydration, handling gas and odor, and addressing nutrient absorption issues and vitamin deficiencies.

5.1 Managing Dehydration

Tips for Staying Hydrated

One of the primary concerns for individuals with an ileostomy is the risk of dehydration. Because the ileostomy bypasses a portion of the small intestine where water absorption occurs, individuals may experience increased fluid loss through their stoma output. To prevent dehydration, it's essential to focus on staying hydrated throughout the day. Here are some tips:

Drink plenty of fluids: Aim to drink at least eight glasses of water per day, or more if you are physically active or in a hot environment. Water is the best choice for hydration, but you can also include other beverages like herbal tea, diluted fruit juice, or electrolyte solutions.

Monitor urine output: Pay attention to the color and frequency of your urine. Pale yellow urine indicates adequate hydration, while dark yellow urine may signal dehydration. Aim for clear to light yellow urine throughout the day.

Consume electrolytes: In addition to water, electrolytes play a crucial role in maintaining hydration. Include foods rich in potassium, sodium, and magnesium in your diet, such as bananas, potatoes, avocados, spinach, and nuts. You can also drink electrolyte-rich beverages or use oral rehydration solutions as recommended by your healthcare provider.

Limit diuretics: Some beverages, such as caffeinated drinks and alcohol, can increase urine output and contribute to dehydration. Limit your intake of these beverages and opt for hydrating alternatives instead.

Monitor stoma output: Pay attention to the consistency and volume of your stoma output. If you notice a significant increase in output or if it becomes watery, you may need to increase your fluid intake to prevent dehydration.

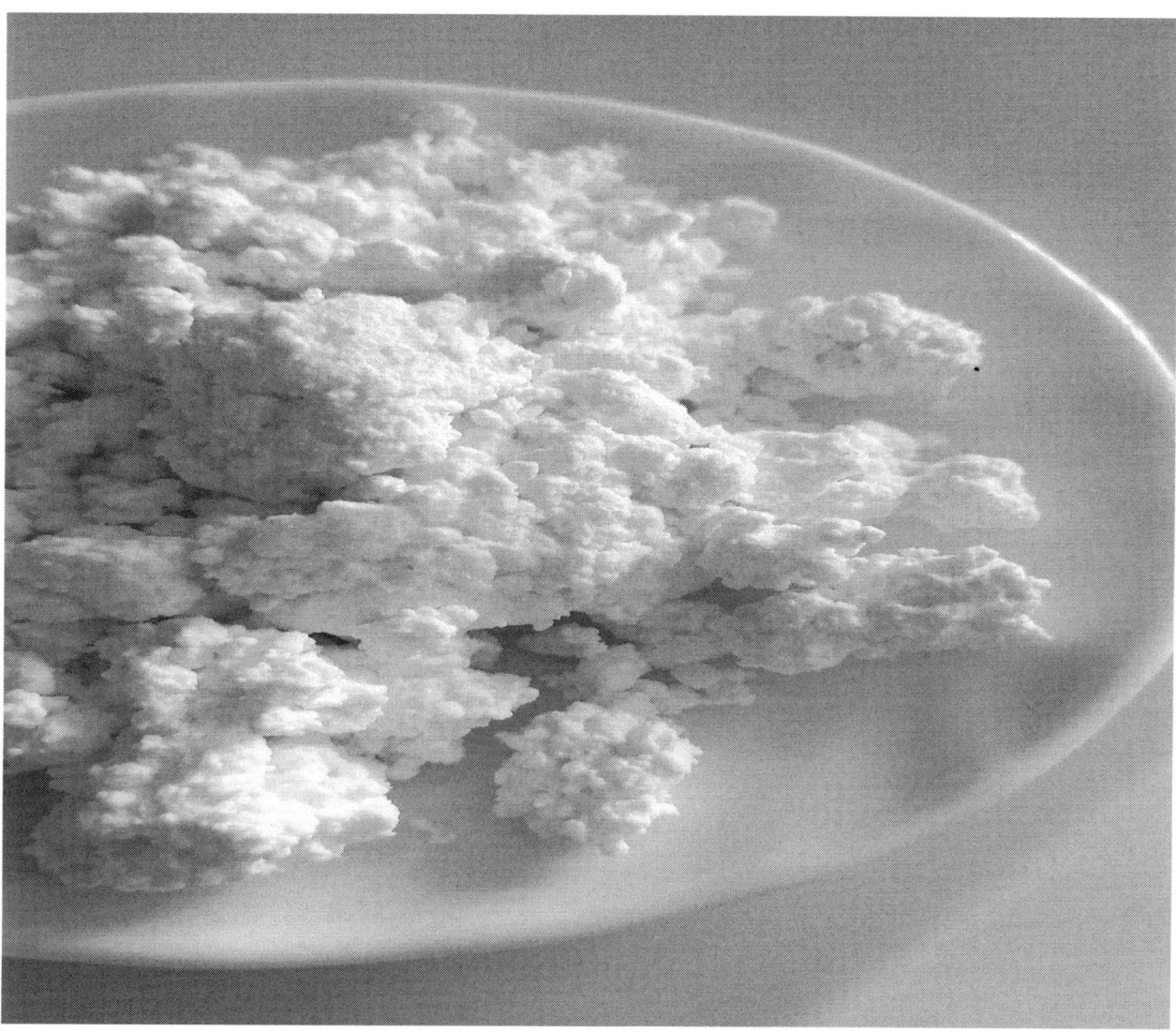

5.2 Handling Gas and Odor: Foods to Minimize Odor and Bloating

Gas and odor are common concerns for individuals with an ileostomy, but certain dietary modifications can help minimize these issues. Here are some tips for managing gas and odor:

Avoid gas-producing foods: Some foods are known to cause excess gas, which can lead to bloating and increased odor in stoma output. These include beans, cabbage, broccoli, onions, and carbonated beverages. Limit your intake of these foods or try alternative cooking methods, such as steaming or baking, to make them easier to digest.

Chew food thoroughly: Properly chewing your food can help reduce the amount of air you swallow, which can contribute to gas and bloating. Take your time to chew each bite thoroughly before swallowing.

Eat smaller, more frequent meals: Large meals can put pressure on your digestive system and lead to increased gas production. Instead, try eating smaller meals throughout the day to help manage gas and bloating.

Experiment with probiotics: Probiotics are beneficial bacteria that can help improve digestion and reduce gas and bloating. Consider incorporating probiotic-rich foods into your diet, such as yogurt, kefir, sauerkraut, and kimchi, or talk to your healthcare provider about taking a probiotic supplement.

Stay hydrated: Dehydration can exacerbate digestive issues, including gas and bloating. Make sure to stay hydrated by drinking plenty of fluids throughout the day.

5.3 Addressing Nutrient Absorption Issues and Vitamin Deficiencies

Due to the altered anatomy of an ileostomy, individuals may experience difficulties with nutrient absorption, leading to vitamin deficiencies. It's essential to address these issues through dietary modifications and, if necessary, supplementation. Here are some strategies for addressing nutrient absorption issues and vitamin deficiencies:

Focus on nutrient-dense foods: Choose foods that are rich in essential nutrients to maximize your intake. Include a variety of fruits, vegetables, whole grains, lean proteins, and healthy fats in your diet to ensure you're getting a wide range of vitamins and minerals.

Consider vitamin supplementation: Depending on your individual needs and the extent of nutrient malabsorption, your healthcare provider may recommend vitamin supplements to prevent deficiencies. Common supplements for individuals with an ileostomy include vitamin B12, vitamin D, calcium, and iron.

Monitor vitamin levels: Regular blood tests can help monitor your vitamin levels and detect any deficiencies early on. Work with your healthcare provider to develop a plan for monitoring and addressing any deficiencies that arise.

Be mindful of fat absorption: Some individuals with an ileostomy may have difficulty absorbing fats, which are essential for the absorption of fat-soluble vitamins (A, D, E, and K). Choose healthy fats, such as olive oil, avocados, nuts, and seeds, and consider taking a digestive enzyme supplement to aid in fat digestion.

CHAPTER 6: ILEOSTOMY-FRIENDLY DIET

BREAKFAST RECIPES

Low-Fiber Pancakes

Prep Time: 10 minutes
Cooking Time: 12 minutes

Ingredients:

- 1 cup refined flour
- 1 tablespoon sugar
- 1 teaspoon baking powder
- 1/2 teaspoon salt
- 1 cup lactose-free milk
- 1 egg
- 2 tablespoons olive oil

Instructions:

- In a mixing bowl, combine flour, sugar, baking powder, and salt.
- In a separate bowl, whisk together milk, egg, and olive oil.
- Gradually add the wet ingredients to the dry ingredients, stirring until just combined.
- Heat a non-stick pan over medium heat and lightly grease with olive oil.
- Pour 1/4 cup of batter onto the pan for each pancake and cook until bubbles form on the surface.
- Flip the pancakes and cook until golden brown on both sides.
- Serve warm with a drizzle of maple syrup or your favorite topping.

Banana Oat Pancakes

Prep Time: 8 minutes
Cooking Time: 10 minutes

Ingredients:
- 2 ripe bananas
- 1 cup rolled oats
- 2 eggs
- 1/2 teaspoon baking powder
- Pinch of salt

Instructions:
- Mash the ripe bananas in a mixing bowl until smooth.
- Add rolled oats, eggs, baking powder, and a pinch of salt to the mashed bananas. Mix until well combined.
- Heat a non-stick skillet over medium heat and lightly grease with cooking spray or oil.
- Pour pancake batter onto the skillet to form pancakes of desired size.
- Cook until bubbles form on the surface, then flip and cook until golden brown on both sides.
- Serve warm with toppings of your choice, such as sliced fruit or a drizzle of honey.

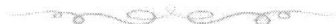

Egg and Spinach Muffins

Prep Time: 7 minutes
Cooking Time: 15 minutes

Ingredients:
- 6 eggs
- 1 cup chopped spinach
- Salt to taste

Instructions:
- Preheat the oven to 350°F (175°C) and grease a muffin tin with cooking spray or oil.
- In a mixing bowl, beat the eggs and season with salt.
- Stir in the chopped spinach until evenly distributed.
- Pour the egg and spinach mixture into the prepared muffin tin, filling each cup about 3/4 full.
- Bake in the preheated oven for 15-20 minutes, or until the muffins are set and lightly golden on top.
- Allow to cool slightly before removing from the muffin tin. Serve warm or at room temperature.

Greek Yogurt Parfait

Prep Time: 5 minutes

Ingredients:
- 1 cup Greek yogurt
- 1/2 cup low-fiber fruits (such as berries)
- 1/4 cup granola

Instructions:
- In a serving glass or bowl, layer Greek yogurt, low-fiber fruits, and granola.
- Repeat the layers until the glass or bowl is filled.
- Serve immediately for a delicious and satisfying breakfast.

Smoothie Bowl

Prep Time: 7 minutes

Ingredients:
- 2 ripe bananas
- 1/2 cup mixed berries (such as strawberries, blueberries, raspberries)
- 1 cup spinach leaves
- 1/2 cup almond milk (or any milk of choice)
- Optional toppings: sliced fruit, shredded coconut, granola, chia seeds

Instructions:
- In a blender, combine bananas, mixed berries, spinach leaves, and almond milk.
- Blend until smooth and creamy, adding more almond milk if needed to reach desired consistency.
- Pour the smoothie into a bowl.
- Top with sliced fruit, shredded coconut, granola, or chia seeds, if desired.
- Enjoy with a spoon for a refreshing and nutritious breakfast.

Scrambled Eggs with Avocado

Prep Time: 3 minutes
Cooking Time: 6 minutes

Ingredients:
- 2 eggs
- 1/2 ripe avocado, sliced
- Salt to taste

Instructions:
- Crack the eggs into a bowl and beat until well mixed.
- Heat a non-stick skillet over medium heat and lightly grease with cooking spray or oil.
- Pour the beaten eggs into the skillet and cook, stirring gently, until they start to set.
- Season with salt and pepper to taste.
- Once the eggs are cooked to your liking, transfer them to a plate.
- Serve with sliced avocado on top for a creamy and satisfying breakfast.

Quinoa Breakfast Bowl

Prep Time: 4 minutes
Cooking Time (if pre-cooked): 0 minutes
Cooking Time (if not pre-cooked): 25 minutes

Ingredients:
- 1/2 cup cooked quinoa
- 1/2 cup cooked apples (cooked with cinnamon and a touch of honey)
- Optional toppings: sliced almonds, raisins, a drizzle of honey

Instructions:
- In a bowl, combine cooked quinoa and cooked apples.
- Stir until well mixed.
- Top with sliced almonds, raisins, and a drizzle of honey, if desired.
- Serve warm for a nutritious and flavorful breakfast.

Cottage Cheese with Peach Slices

Prep Time: 5 minutes

Ingredients:
- 1/2 cup cottage cheese
- 1 ripe peach, peeled and sliced

Instructions:
- In a serving bowl, place the cottage cheese.
- Top with the peeled and sliced peach.
- Enjoy as it is or drizzle with a touch of honey for added sweetness, if desired.

Turkey and Cheese Roll-Ups

Prep Time: 5 minutes

Ingredients:
- 4 slices turkey breast
- 2 slices cheese (such as cheddar or Swiss)

Instructions:
- Lay turkey breast slices flat on a clean surface.
- Place a slice of cheese on each turkey slice.
- Roll up tightly.
- Serve as a low-fiber, protein-rich breakfast option.

Almond Butter and Banana Toast

Prep Time: 5 minutes
Cooking Time: 2-3 minutes (for toasting the bread)

Ingredients:
- 2 slices whole-grain bread
- 2 tablespoons smooth almond butter
- 1 ripe banana, sliced

Instructions:
- Toast the slices of whole-grain bread until golden brown.
- Spread smooth almond butter evenly over each slice of toast.
- Arrange sliced banana on top of the almond butter.
- Serve immediately for a delicious and filling breakfast.

Yogurt and Berry Smoothie

Prep Time: 5 minutes

Ingredients:
- 1 cup Greek yogurt
- 1/2 cup mixed berries (such as strawberries, blueberries, raspberries)
- 1/2 cup coconut water
- Optional: honey or maple syrup to taste

Instructions:

- In a blender, combine Greek yogurt, mixed berries, and coconut water.
- Blend until smooth and creamy.
- If desired, strain the smoothie to remove seeds for easier digestion.
- Taste and add honey or maple syrup if desired for sweetness.
- Pour into a glass and serve immediately as a refreshing breakfast smoothie.

Egg White Omelett

Prep Time: 5 minutes
Cooking Time: 5-7 minutes

Ingredients:
- 4 egg whites
- 1/4 cup diced tomatoes
- 1/4 cup shredded cheese (such as mozzarella or feta)
- Salt to taste
- Cooking spray or oil for greasing the pan

Instructions:
- In a bowl, whisk together egg whites until frothy.
- Heat a non-stick skillet over medium heat and lightly grease with cooking spray or oil.
- Pour the whisked egg whites into the skillet.
- Sprinkle diced, peeled, and seedless tomatoes evenly over the egg whites.
- Cook until the edges start to set, then sprinkle shredded cheese over one half of the omelette.
- Using a spatula, fold the omelette in half and continue cooking until the cheese is melted and the eggs are cooked through.
- Season with salt to taste.
- Slide the omelette onto a plate and serve hot.

Cinnamon Apple Porridge

Prep Time: 5 minutes
Cooking Time: 5-7 minutes

Ingredients:
- 1/2 cup quick oats or instant oats
- 1 cup water or milk (almond milk or any milk of choice)
- 1/2 apple, peeled and finely diced
- 1/2 teaspoon ground cinnamon
- 1 tablespoon maple syrup (optional)

- ## Instructions:
- In a small saucepan, bring water or milk to a simmer over medium heat.
- Stir in the quick oats or instant oats and the peeled, finely diced apple.
- Reduce heat to low and cook, stirring occasionally, for 5-7 minutes or until the oats are cooked and the porridge has thickened, and the apple is very soft.
- Stir in ground cinnamon and maple syrup, if using.
- Remove from heat and let it sit for a minute.
- Transfer the porridge to a bowl and serve warm.

Smoked Salmon and Cream Cheese Bagel

Prep Time: 5 minutes
Cooking Time: 2-3 minutes (for toasting the bagel)

Ingredients:
- 1 plain bagel, sliced and toasted
- 2 ounces smoked salmon
- 2 tablespoons cream cheese
- Optional: peeled and thinly sliced cucumber

Instructions:
- Spread cream cheese on each half of the toasted plain bagel.
- Layer smoked salmon on top of the cream cheese.
- Add peeled and thinly sliced cucumber, if desired.
- Serve immediately for a delicious and satisfying breakfast.

Rice Cake with Peanut Butter and Sliced Banana

Prep Time: 5 minutes

Ingredients:
- 1 rice cake
- 1 tablespoon smooth peanut butter
- 1/2 ripe banana, sliced

Instructions:
- Spread smooth peanut butter evenly over the rice cake.
- Arrange sliced banana on top of the peanut butter.
- Serve immediately for a quick and satisfying breakfast.

Mango Coconut Yogurt Bowl

Prep Time: 5 minutes

Ingredients:
- 1 cup Greek yogurt (lactose-free if necessary)
- 1/2 ripe mango, peeled and diced
- 1 tablespoon finely shredded or desiccated coconut
- Optional: honey or maple syrup to taste

Instructions:

- In a serving bowl, place Greek yogurt.
- Top with peeled and diced mango and finely shredded or desiccated coconut.
- Drizzle with honey or maple syrup if desired for added sweetness.
- Serve immediately for a tropical-inspired breakfast.

Egg and Cheese Breakfast Quesadilla

Prep Time: 5 minutes
Cooking Time: 6-8 minutes

Ingredients:
- 2 whole-grain tortillas
- 2 eggs, scrambled
- 1/4 cup shredded cheese (such as cheddar or Monterey Jack)
- Salsa for serving

Instructions:
- Heat a non-stick skillet over medium heat.
- Place one tortilla in the skillet and top with scrambled eggs and shredded cheese.
- Place the second tortilla on top.
- Cook for 2-3 minutes on each side, or until the tortillas are golden brown and the cheese is melted.
- Slice into wedges and serve with salsa for dipping.

Vanilla Protein Shake

Prep Time: 5 minutes

Ingredients:
- 1 scoop vanilla protein powder (low-fiber and low-additive)
- 1 cup almond milk (or any milk of choice)
- Ice cubes

Instructions:
- In a blender, combine vanilla protein powder and almond milk.
- Add ice cubes to the blender.
- Blend until smooth and creamy.
- Pour into a glass and serve immediately as a quick and easy breakfast on the go.

Cheddar Cheese and Tomato Toast

Prep Time: 5 minutes
Cooking Time: 7 minutes

Ingredients:
- 2 slices low-fiber bread, toasted
- 1/2 cup shredded cheddar cheese
- 1 medium tomato, thinly sliced
- Salt to taste

Instructions:
- Preheat the oven to 350°F (175°C).
- Place the toasted bread slices on a baking sheet.
- Sprinkle shredded cheddar cheese evenly over each slice of toast.
- Arrange tomato slices on top of the cheese.
- Season with salt to taste.
- Bake in the preheated oven for 5-7 minutes, or until the cheese is melted and bubbly.
- Serve hot as a simple yet satisfying breakfast.

Blueberry Almond Smoothie

Prep Time: 5 minutes

Ingredients:
- 1 cup almond milk (or any milk of choice)
- 1/4 cup frozen blueberries (well-blended)
- 1 tablespoon almond butter
- 1/2 teaspoon ground cinnamon

Instructions:
- In a blender, combine almond milk, frozen blueberries, almond butter, and ground cinnamon.
- Blend until smooth and creamy.
- Pour into a glass and serve immediately as a nutritious breakfast drink.

LUNCH RECIPES

Quinoa Salad with Grilled Chicken

Ingredients:
- 1 cup quinoa (or substitute with white rice if quinoa is not well-tolerated)
- 2 cups water
- 1 grilled chicken breast, diced
- 1 cucumber, peeled, seeded, and diced
- 1/4 cup chopped parsley (optional)
- 2 tablespoons olive oil
- Salt to taste

Directions:
- Rinse quinoa under cold water. Cook quinoa in water according to package instructions (usually about 15 minutes).
- In a large bowl, combine cooked quinoa, diced chicken, peeled and seeded cucumber, and parsley.
- Drizzle olive oil over the salad and season with salt. Toss to combine.
- Serve immediately or chill in the refrigerator for later.

Turkey and Avocado Wrap

Ingredients:
- 1 large refined flour tortilla
- 4 slices turkey breast
- 1/4 avocado, thinly sliced
- 2 tablespoons finely shredded lettuce (optional)
- 2 tablespoons smooth hummus

Directions:
- Lay the tortilla flat on a clean surface.
- Spread smooth hummus evenly over the tortilla.
- Layer turkey slices, thinly sliced avocado, and finely shredded lettuce (if using) on top of the hummus.
- Roll the tortilla tightly and slice it in half.
- Serve immediately for a quick and satisfying meal.

Salmon and Quinoa Bowl

Prep Time: 10 minutes
Cooking Time: 20-25 minutes

Ingredients:
- 1 cup cooked quinoa
- 1 grilled salmon fillet, flaked
- 1 cup well-cooked broccoli florets
- 1/4 cup lightly steamed shredded carrots
- 2 tablespoons low-sodium soy sauce
- 1 tablespoon sesame oil

Directions:
- In a bowl, layer cooked quinoa, flaked salmon, steamed broccoli, and shredded carrots.
- In a small bowl, whisk together soy sauce and sesame oil. Drizzle over the quinoa bowl before serving.

Egg Salad Lettuce Wraps

Ingredients:
- 4 hard-boiled eggs, chopped
- 2 tablespoons Greek yogurt
- 1 tablespoon Dijon mustard
- 1/4 cup diced celery
- Salt to taste
- Butter lettuce leaves

Directions:
- Cook Quinoa (or Rice): Rinse 1/2 cup of quinoa under cold water. Combine with 1 cup of water in a pot and bring to a boil. Reduce to a simmer, cover, and cook for about 15 minutes until water is absorbed and quinoa is tender. If using rice, follow package instructions.
- Grill Salmon: Preheat grill to medium-high heat. Season the salmon fillet with salt and a little oil. Grill for about 4-5 minutes on each side until cooked through. Allow to cool slightly and then flake.
- Steam Broccoli: Steam 1 cup of broccoli florets until very soft, about 7-10 minutes.
- Steam Carrots: Lightly steam 1/4 cup shredded carrots for about 3-5 minutes.
- Assemble Bowl: In a bowl, layer cooked quinoa (or rice), flaked salmon, steamed broccoli, and steamed shredded carrots.
- Prepare Dressing: In a small bowl, whisk together 2 tablespoons low-sodium soy sauce and 1 tablespoon sesame oil. Drizzle over the bowl before serving.

Tuna and White Bean Salad

Ingredients:
- 1 can tuna, drained
- 1 can white beans, rinsed and drained
- 1/4 cup diced red onion
- 1/4 cup chopped parsley
- 2 tablespoons olive oil
- 1 tablespoon lemon juice
- Salt to taste

Directions:
- In a large bowl, combine tuna, white beans, diced red onion, and chopped parsley.
- Drizzle olive oil and lemon juice over the salad. Season with salt.
- Mix well before serving.

Chicken and Vegetable Stir-Fry

Ingredients:
- 1 tablespoon olive oil
- 1 boneless, skinless chicken breast, sliced
- 1 cup sliced bell peppers (optional, omit if you prefer)
- 1 cup sliced zucchini
- 1 cup sliced mushrooms
- 2 tablespoons soy sauce
- 1 tablespoon honey
- Cooked rice for serving

Directions:
- Heat olive oil in a skillet over medium heat. Add sliced chicken breast and cook until browned.
- Add sliced zucchini and mushrooms to the skillet. Cook until vegetables are tender.
- In a small bowl, mix soy sauce and honey. Pour over the chicken and vegetables. Stir to combine.
- Serve the stir-fry over cooked rice.

Mashed Sweet Potatoes with Grilled Shrimp

Ingredients:
- 2 large sweet potatoes, peeled and diced
- 12 large shrimp, peeled and deveined
- 2 tablespoons olive oil
- 1 teaspoon garlic powder
- Salt to taste

Directions:
- Boil sweet potatoes in a pot of water until tender. Drain and mash with a fork.
- Season shrimp with olive oil, garlic powder, and salt. Grill until cooked through.
- Serve grilled shrimp over mashed sweet potatoes.

Spinach and Feta Omelette

Ingredients:
- 2 eggs
- 1/4 cup baby spinach leaves
- 2 tablespoons crumbled feta cheese
- Salt to taste
- Cooking spray

Directions:
- In a bowl, whisk together eggs, spinach, and feta cheese. Season with salt.
- Heat a non-stick skillet over medium heat and coat with cooking spray.
- Pour the egg mixture into the skillet and cook until the edges start to set.
- Flip the omelette and cook until fully set. Fold it in half and serve hot.

Baked Cod with Steamed Vegetables

Ingredients:
- 2 cod fillets
- 1 lemon, sliced
- 1 tablespoon olive oil
- Salt to taste
- Assorted steamed vegetables (e.g., broccoli, carrots, cauliflower)

Directions:
- Preheat the oven to 375°F (190°C). Place cod fillets on a baking sheet lined with parchment paper.
- Drizzle olive oil over the cod fillets and season with salt. Place lemon slices on top.
- Bake for 15-20 minutes or until the fish is cooked through.
- Serve baked cod with steamed vegetables on the side.

Turkey and Vegetable Soup

Ingredients:
- 2 cups diced cooked turkey breast
- 4 cups low-sodium chicken broth
- 1 cup diced carrots
- 1 cup diced celery
- 1 cup diced potatoes
- 1/2 cup diced onion
- 2 cloves garlic, minced
- 1 teaspoon dried thyme
- Salt to taste

Directions:
- In a large pot, combine chicken broth, diced turkey, carrots, celery, potatoes, onion, garlic, and thyme.
- Bring the soup to a boil, then reduce the heat and let it simmer for about 20-25 minutes until vegetables are tender.
- Season with salt before serving.

Shredded Chicken and Brown Rice Bowl

Ingredients:
- 1 cup cooked brown rice
- 1 cup shredded cooked chicken breast
- 1/2 cup steamed green beans
- 1/4 cup diced tomatoes
- 2 tablespoons chopped cilantro
- 1 tablespoon olive oil
- 1 tablespoon lemon juice
- Salt to taste

Directions:
- In a bowl, combine cooked brown rice, shredded chicken breast, steamed green beans, diced tomatoes, and chopped cilantro.
- Drizzle olive oil and lemon juice over the bowl. Season with salt. Mix well and serve.

Tofu and Vegetable Stir-Fry

Ingredients:
- 1 tablespoon sesame oil
- 1 block firm tofu, cubed
- 2 cups mixed vegetables (such as bell peppers, broccoli, carrots)
- 2 tablespoons low-sodium soy sauce
- 1 tablespoon rice vinegar
- 1 teaspoon minced ginger
- 2 cloves garlic, minced
- Cooked brown rice for serving

Directions:
- Heat sesame oil in a large skillet over medium heat. Add cubed tofu and cook until golden brown on all sides.
- Add mixed vegetables, minced ginger, and minced garlic to the skillet. Stir-fry until vegetables are tender.
- In a small bowl, mix soy sauce and rice vinegar. Pour over the tofu and vegetables. Stir to combine.
- Serve the tofu and vegetable stir-fry over cooked brown rice.

Lentil Soup with Spinach

Ingredients:
- 1 cup dried lentils, rinsed
- 4 cups low-sodium vegetable broth
- 1 onion, diced
- 2 carrots, diced
- 2 celery stalks, diced
- 2 cloves garlic, minced
- 2 cups chopped spinach
- 1 teaspoon dried thyme
- Salt to taste

Directions:
- In a large pot, combine lentils, vegetable broth, diced onion, carrots, celery, garlic, and thyme.
- Bring the soup to a boil, then reduce the heat and let it simmer for about 30-35 minutes until the lentils are tender.
- Stir in chopped spinach and cook for an additional 5 minutes until wilted. Season with salt before serving.

Grilled Vegetable Salad

Ingredients:
- 2 zucchinis, sliced lengthwise
- 2 bell peppers, quartered (optional, omit if you prefer)
- 1 eggplant, sliced
- 1 red onion, sliced into rings
- 2 tablespoons olive oil
- 2 tablespoons balsamic vinegar
- Salt to taste

Directions:
- Preheat the grill to medium-high heat. Brush zucchini, (omit bell peppers), eggplant, and red onion with olive oil.
- Grill vegetables for 5-7 minutes per side until tender and grill marks appear.
- Remove from the grill and let them cool slightly. Cut grilled vegetables into bite-sized pieces.
- In a large bowl, toss grilled vegetables with balsamic vinegar. Season with salt. Serve warm or at room temperature.

Miso Soup with Tofu and Seaweed

Ingredients:
- 4 cups low-sodium vegetable broth
- 1/4 cup miso paste
- 1 block firm tofu, cubed
- 2 green onions, sliced
- 2 sheets nori seaweed, torn into small pieces
- 1 teaspoon sesame oil
- Salt to taste

Directions:
- In a pot, bring vegetable broth to a simmer. Whisk in miso paste until dissolved.
- Add cubed tofu, sliced green onions, and torn nori seaweed to the pot. Simmer for 5 minutes.
- Remove from heat and stir in sesame oil.
- Season with salt before serving.

ASIAN RECIPES

Steamed Fish with Ginger and Scallions

Ingredients:
- 2 fish fillets (such as tilapia or cod)
- 2 tablespoons ginger, julienned
- 2 scallions, sliced
- 2 tablespoons soy sauce
- 1 tablespoon sesame oil

Directions:
- Place fish fillets on a plate.
- Scatter ginger and scallions over the fish.
- Steam for 8-10 minutes until fish is cooked.
- Drizzle soy sauce and sesame oil over the fish before serving.

Vegetable Stir-Fry

Ingredients:
- 2 cups mixed vegetables (carrots, broccoli, snap peas)
- 2 tablespoons vegetable oil
- 2 cloves garlic, minced
- 2 tablespoons soy sauce

Directions:
- Heat oil in a pan over medium heat.
- Add garlic and stir-fry for 30 seconds.
- Add mixed vegetables and stir-fry for 3-4 minutes.
- Mix in soy sauce and cook for another 2 minutes.

Ginger Chicken Congee

Ingredients:
- 1 cup rice
- 4 cups chicken broth
- 1 chicken breast, thinly sliced
- 2 tablespoons ginger, minced

Directions:
- Rinse rice and add to a pot with chicken broth.
- Bring to a boil, then reduce heat and simmer for 30 minutes, stirring occasionally.
- Add sliced chicken and ginger, simmer for another 10 minutes until chicken is cooked.

Japanese Omelette (Tamagoyaki)

Ingredients:
- 4 eggs
- 2 tablespoons soy sauce
- 1 tablespoon mirin
- 1 tablespoon sugar

Directions:
- Beat eggs in a bowl and mix in soy sauce, mirin, and sugar.
- Heat a non-stick pan over medium heat and lightly oil.
- Pour a thin layer of egg mixture into the pan and cook until set but still slightly runny.
- Roll the omelette from one end to the other, then push it to the edge of the pan.
- Oil the pan again and pour another thin layer of egg mixture, lifting the rolled omelette to let the new layer flow underneath.
- Repeat until all the egg mixture is used.

Rice Noodle Soup

Ingredients:
- 100g rice noodles
- 4 cups chicken or vegetable broth
- 1 cup sliced mushrooms
- 1 cup baby spinach

Directions:
- Cook rice noodles according to package instructions, then drain and set aside.
- In a pot, bring broth to a simmer and add mushrooms.
- Cook for 5 minutes, then add spinach.
- Simmer for another 2 minutes, then add cooked rice noodles.

PORTUGUESE RECIPES

Bacalhau à Brás (Portuguese Salt Cod Hash)

Ingredients:
- 500g salt cod, soaked and shredded
- 500g potatoes, thinly sliced into matchsticks
- 2 onions, thinly sliced (optional)
- 4 eggs
- Olive oil

Directions:
- Fry potatoes in olive oil until golden and crispy, then set aside.
- In the same pan, fry onions until soft.
- Add shredded salt cod to the pan and cook for a few minutes.
- Add fried potatoes to the pan and mix well.
- Crack eggs into the pan and scramble until cooked.

Caldo Verde (Portuguese Green Soup)

Ingredients:
- 4 cups chicken or vegetable broth
- 2 potatoes, diced
- 1 onion, finely chopped
- 2 cups kale, thinly sliced
- Olive oil

Directions:
- In a pot, heat olive oil and sauté onions until translucent.
- Add diced potatoes and chicken broth, then simmer until potatoes are tender.
- Mash some of the potatoes to thicken the soup.
- Add sliced kale and cook until wilted.

Grilled Sardines

Ingredients:
- 8 fresh sardines, gutted and cleaned
- Olive oil

Directions:
- Preheat the grill to medium-high heat.
- Brush sardines with olive oil.
- Grill sardines for 3-4 minutes on each side until cooked through.

Portuguese Chicken and Rice

Ingredients:
- 4 chicken thighs, bone-in and skin-on
- 2 cups white rice
- 4 cups chicken broth
- 1 onion, finely chopped(optional)

Directions:
- Season chicken thighs with salt and pepper.
- In a pot, heat olive oil and brown chicken thighs on both sides.
- Remove chicken from the pot and sauté onions until soft.
- Add rice, chicken broth, and browned chicken thighs to the pot.

Portuguese Custard Tarts (Pastéis de Nata)

Ingredients:
- 1 sheet puff pastry, thawed
- 2 cups milk
- 4 egg yolks
- 1/2 cup sugar
- 2 tablespoons cornstarch
- 1 teaspoon vanilla extract

Directions:
- Preheat the oven to 220°C (425°F).
- Roll out puff pastry and cut into squares to fit into muffin tins.
- In a saucepan, heat milk until steaming but not boiling.
- In a bowl, whisk together egg yolks, sugar, cornstarch, and vanilla extract until smooth.
- Slowly pour hot milk into the egg mixture, whisking constantly.

SPANISH RECIPES

Spanish Tortilla (Tortilla Española)

Ingredients:
- 4 potatoes, thinly sliced
- 1 onion, thinly sliced(optional)
- 6 eggs
- Olive oil

Directions:
- Heat olive oil in a non-stick skillet over medium heat.
- Add potatoes and onions to the skillet and cook until potatoes are tender.
- In a bowl, beat eggs and season with salt and pepper.
- Pour eggs over the potatoes and onions in the skillet.

Gazpacho

Ingredients:
- 4 ripe tomatoes, chopped
- 1 cucumber, peeled and chopped
- 2 cloves garlic, minced
- 2 tablespoons olive oil
- 2 tablespoons red wine vinegar

Directions:
- Blend tomatoes, cucumber, and garlic until smooth.
- Stir in olive oil and red wine vinegar.

Spanish Rice with Shrimp

Ingredients:
- 1 cup rice
- 2 cups chicken broth
- 2 cloves garlic, minced
- Olive oil

Directions:
- In a pot, heat olive oil and sauté garlic until softened.
- Add rice and cook for 1-2 minutes.
- Stir in chicken broth.
- Bring to a boil, then reduce heat and simmer until rice is cooked.

Patatas Bravas

Ingredients:
- 4 potatoes, diced
- Olive oil
- 1/4 cup mayonnaise

Directions:
- Preheat the oven to 200°C (400°F).
- Toss diced potatoes with olive oil and spread on a baking sheet.
- Bake for 20-25 minutes until potatoes are golden and crispy.
- Serve with mayonnaise.

Spanish Chicken Paella

Ingredients:
- 2 chicken breasts, diced
- 1 onion, finely chopped
- 2 cloves garlic, minced
- 1 red bell pepper, diced
- 1 cup rice
- 2 cups chicken broth
- Olive oil

Directions:
- In a paella pan or large skillet, heat olive oil and cook chicken until browned.
- Remove chicken from the pan and set aside.
- In the same pan, sauté onions, garlic, and red bell pepper until softened.
- Stir in rice and cook for 1-2 minutes.
- Add chicken broth to the pan, then bring to a boil.
- Reduce heat and simmer until rice is cooked.

ITALIAN RECIPES

Caprese Salad

Ingredients:
- 2 large tomatoes, sliced
- 200g fresh mozzarella cheese, sliced
- Fresh basil leaves
- Olive oil

Directions:
- Arrange tomato and mozzarella slices on a serving platter.
- Tuck fresh basil leaves between the slices.
- Drizzle with olive oil.

Pasta Primavera

Ingredients:
- 250g pasta (spaghetti or penne)
- 2 cups mixed vegetables (zucchini, cherry tomatoes)
- 2 cloves garlic, minced
- Olive oil

Directions:
- Cook pasta according to package instructions.
- In a pan, heat olive oil and sauté garlic until fragrant.
- Add mixed vegetables to the pan and cook until tender.
- Toss cooked pasta with the vegetables.

Chicken Piccata

Prep Time: 10 minutes
Cooking Time: 10 minutes

Ingredients:
- 4 chicken breasts, pounded thin
- 1/2 cup flour
- 2 tablespoons olive oil

Directions:

- Dredge chicken breasts in flour, shaking off excess.
- Heat olive oil in a skillet over medium-high heat.
- Cook chicken breasts for 3-4 minutes on each side until golden brown and cooked through.
- Optionally, season with a small amount of salt.

Minestrone Soup

Prep Time: 10 minutes
Cooking Time: 25 minutes

Ingredients:
- 2 carrots, diced
- 1 clove garlic, minced (optional and use in moderation)
- 1 can smooth tomato sauce (or diced tomatoes, sieved to remove seeds and skins)
- 4 cups vegetable broth
- 1 cup small pasta (macaroni or shells)
- 2 tablespoons olive oil

Directions:
- In a pot, heat olive oil over medium heat and sauté finely chopped onions, diced carrots, and minced garlic (if using) until they are softened and well-cooked (about 5-7 minutes).
- Add smooth tomato sauce (or sieved diced tomatoes) and vegetable broth to the pot.
- Bring to a boil, then add the small pasta.
- Reduce heat and simmer until the pasta is fully cooked and the vegetables are tender (about 10-15 minutes).
- Serve hot.

Tiramisu

Prep Time: 20 minutes
Chilling Time: At least 4 hours (preferably overnight)

Ingredients:
- 250g mascarpone cheese
- 1 cup heavy cream (use a lighter cream if high fat is an issue)
- 1/2 cup powdered sugar
- 1 teaspoon vanilla extract
- Ladyfinger biscuits (or soft sponge cake)
- Decaffeinated coffee (or milk)

Directions:

- In a bowl, whisk together mascarpone cheese, heavy cream, powdered sugar, and vanilla extract until smooth and creamy.
- Dip ladyfinger biscuits (or pieces of soft sponge cake) into decaffeinated coffee (or milk) and layer them in a serving dish.
- Spread half of the mascarpone mixture over the soaked ladyfingers.
- Repeat layers with remaining ladyfingers and mascarpone mixture.
- Cover and refrigerate tiramisu for at least 4 hours or overnight.

BONUS

MEAL PLAN

Week 1:

Day 1:
Breakfast: Oatmeal with banana slices and a dollop of honey.
Lunch: Grilled chicken breast with steamed carrots and mashed potatoes.
Dinner: Baked salmon with quinoa and steamed green beans.

Day 2:
Breakfast: Scrambled eggs with spinach and whole grain toast.
Lunch: Turkey and avocado wrap with lettuce and tomato.
Dinner: Stir-fried tofu with mixed vegetables and brown rice.

Day 3:
Breakfast: Yogurt parfait with granola and berries.
Lunch: Vegetable soup with a side of whole grain crackers.
Dinner: Roast beef with roasted sweet potatoes and steamed broccoli.

Day 4:
Breakfast: Smoothie made with spinach, banana, almond milk, and protein powder.
Lunch: Grilled shrimp salad with mixed greens, cucumber, and balsamic vinaigrette.
Dinner: Baked chicken thighs with roasted Brussels sprouts and quinoa.

Day 5:
Breakfast: Cottage cheese with sliced peaches and a sprinkle of cinnamon.
Lunch: Quinoa salad with black beans, corn, cherry tomatoes, and avocado.
Dinner: Pork tenderloin with roasted carrots and mashed cauliflower.

Day 6:
Breakfast: Whole grain toast with almond butter and sliced strawberries.
Lunch: Lentil soup with a side of whole grain bread.
Dinner: Grilled tilapia with steamed asparagus and wild rice.

Day 7:
Breakfast: Greek yogurt with honey and chopped almonds.
Lunch: Chicken Caesar salad with homemade dressing and croutons.
Dinner: Turkey meatballs with zucchini noodles and marinara sauce.

Week 2:

Day 8:
Breakfast: Cottage cheese with sliced peaches and a sprinkle of cinnamon.
Lunch: Quinoa salad with black beans, corn, cherry tomatoes, and avocado.
Dinner: Pork tenderloin with roasted carrots and mashed cauliflower.

Day 9:
Breakfast: Smoothie made with spinach, banana, almond milk, and protein powder.
Lunch: Grilled shrimp salad with mixed greens, cucumber, and balsamic vinaigrette.
Dinner: Baked chicken thighs with roasted Brussels sprouts and quinoa.

Day 10:
Breakfast: Oatmeal with banana slices and a dollop of honey.
Lunch: Grilled chicken breast with steamed carrots and mashed potatoes.
Dinner: Baked salmon with quinoa and steamed green beans.

Day 11:
Breakfast: Whole grain toast with almond butter and sliced strawberries.
Lunch: Lentil soup with a side of whole grain bread.
Dinner: Grilled tilapia with steamed asparagus and wild rice.

Day 12:
Breakfast: Greek yogurt with honey and chopped almonds.
Lunch: Chicken Caesar salad with homemade dressing and croutons.
Dinner: Turkey meatballs with zucchini noodles and marinara sauce.

Day 13:
Breakfast: Poached eggs with sautéed spinach and whole grain toast.
Lunch: Quinoa and black bean stuffed bell peppers with a side of avocado.
Dinner: Baked turkey breast with roasted sweet potatoes and steamed broccoli.

Day 14:
Breakfast: Whole grain toast with mashed avocado and sliced tomatoes.
Lunch: Turkey and cranberry wrap with mixed greens.
Dinner: Baked tofu with stir-fried bok choy and brown rice.

Week 3:

Day 15:
Breakfast: Overnight oats with almond milk, chia seeds, and sliced strawberries.
Lunch: Grilled vegetable and hummus wrap with a side of baby carrots.
Dinner: Baked cod with lemon, served with steamed green beans and quinoa.

Day 16:
Breakfast: Whole grain pancakes with Greek yogurt and blueberries.
Lunch: Spinach and feta salad with roasted chickpeas and a lemon-tahini dressing.
Dinner: Beef stir-fry with bell peppers, snap peas, and brown rice.

Day 17:
Breakfast: Smoothie bowl with blended mango, pineapple, and coconut milk, topped with shredded coconut and sliced almonds.
Lunch: Tomato basil soup with a side of whole grain bread.
Dinner: Grilled chicken skewers with bell peppers and onions, served with couscous.

Day 18:
Breakfast: Poached eggs with sautéed spinach and whole grain toast.
Lunch: Quinoa and black bean stuffed bell peppers with a side of avocado.
Dinner: Baked turkey breast with roasted sweet potatoes and steamed broccoli.

Day 19:
Breakfast: Cottage cheese with sliced peaches and a drizzle of honey.
Lunch: Lentil salad with cucumbers, tomatoes, and a lemon-herb vinaigrette.
Dinner: Grilled salmon with roasted asparagus and wild rice.

Day 20:
Breakfast: Whole grain toast with mashed avocado and sliced tomatoes.
Lunch: Turkey and cranberry wrap with mixed greens.
Dinner: Baked tofu with stir-fried bok choy and brown rice.

Day 21:
Breakfast: Greek yogurt parfait with granola and mixed berries.
Lunch: Chicken and vegetable stir-fry with teriyaki sauce and quinoa.
Dinner: Beef kebabs with grilled zucchini and couscous.

CONCLUSION

Adjusting to life with an ileostomy can be a significant transition, often accompanied by dietary concerns and uncertainties. For individuals navigating this journey, a well-curated ileostomy diet cookbook can serve as a valuable resource, offering not only recipes but also insights into crafting a nourishing and enjoyable diet tailored to specific needs.

Following ileostomy surgery, individuals may face various challenges related to diet and nutrition. The altered digestive system can affect nutrient absorption, leading to concerns about maintaining adequate levels of essential vitamins and minerals. Moreover, certain foods may trigger digestive discomfort or exacerbate symptoms such as diarrhea or dehydration. Getting through these challenges requires a detailed approach, one that prioritizes nutrient density, digestive tolerance, and culinary satisfaction.

ILEOSTOMY DIET COOKBOOK FOR BEGINNERS serves as a guidance amidst the dietary uncertainties. Unlike generic cookbooks, which may not address the unique needs of individuals with an ileostomy, this **COOKBOOK** is tailored to provide practical solutions and culinary inspiration. From simple yet nutritious meal ideas to special recipes that accommodate dietary restrictions, this cookbook will empower you to explore a diverse range of flavors and ingredients while prioritizing digestive health and overall well-being.

Printed in Great Britain
by Amazon